Table of Contents

REAL TALK

WITH

REAL FIT PROS

THE INSIDER SCOOP ON ACHIEVING YOUR FITNESS GOALS

BY JONATHAN LAUTERMILCH AND MARC ZALMANOFF

Published by

Smart Shark Publishing

PROLOGUE

*It is a shame for a man to grow old, without seeing the beauty
and strength of which his body is capable*

—Socrates

Fitness means a lot of different things to a lot of ***not so
different people***. For some, it's how they look and how
they view themselves. For others, it's how they move and
how they feel. And for many, most importantly, it's adding
years of quality existence to their lives. Whatever fitness
means to you, we want you to know that all things are
possible when you combine three simple concepts.

One: Information Leads to TRANSFORMATION

When you arm yourself with the right information regarding
your health and fitness, you are then able to not only take
action, but action that leads to you experiencing REAL
CHANGE. This is the kind of change that leads to a level of
belief that once you experience it, you simply just can't go
back to the way things were.

To us, fitness is a life-long pursuit not only achieved one
time, but accomplished over and over again. This is exactly
what you will learn by reading the stories from real fit pros

who have not just learned how to do it for themselves, but have become masters at helping others do the same.

Two: How You Do One Thing is How You Do EVERYTHING

We tend to put different areas of our lives into categories that all get treated differently. Some get all of our attention, while others get little to no attention.

Those areas are:
- Your fitness (your health)
- Your faith (the faith you have in yourself)
- Your family (chosen and not by choice)
- Your finances (your career)

Most people spend their entire lives with fitness being the bottom of their focus and wonder why they struggle in their careers, their marriages, and their confidence in themselves. We're here to challenge that very way of doing life by making fitness the FIRST area you focus on, which serves as the bedrock to building and growing in other areas. How we operate in one area determines how we operate in others. How we do one thing will always be how we do everything.

Three: Alignment Over Assignment

Become extremely intentional about who you surround yourself with when it comes to doing this thing we call *life*.

We (The Fit Pro Bros Jonathan Lautermilch and Marc Zalmanoff) have been in the fitness industry helping thousands of people over the past thirty years combined. We notice those who have a strong community to lean on are the ones who make fitness part of their lifestyle, while those who try to go it alone almost always fall off at some point.

The reason, we believe, is we become the sum of the five people we spend the most time with. If you hang out with five unhealthy people, you'll most definitely be the sixth. But, if you hang out with five healthy people, you'll also most definitely become the sixth. Part of finding your group to grow with on your fitness journey is clearly defining your core values. Those values will help you identify the right people to surround yourself with, so you can flourish not only with your health and fitness, but in every other area of your life as well.

As you'll read in this book, you'll learn one of our core values is Professional. For us, this means, "We understand that in order to lead others we must first lead ourselves." We can proudly say the authors in this book are true leaders in every sense of the word in terms of leading from the front for their clients and followers.

The purpose of this book is to truly help you get what you're worth in every area of your life through getting the right information, the right mindset, and the right community to support you along the way.

We look forward to helping you get what you're worth and can't wait to see you on the other side.

CHAPTER ONE:
The Five Words That Changed My Life

by Victor Fernandes

For once, I heard precisely what I needed to hear.

"Can you afford not to?" the health and fitness coach sitting across from me asked. I hadn't been asked that before, which made it easy for me to say no to previous coaches because, well, I couldn't afford it.

Those five simple yet powerful words more than a decade ago hit me like a ton of bricks falling on my head, but still weighed me down less than weighing nearly 250 lbs. and in the worst shape of my life mentally, emotionally, and physically.

I was finally ready to listen. I *needed* to listen.

My newborn son, Zachary, needed me to listen. And I didn't know it at the time, but my wife Shelly needed me to listen too. She was a few months away from being diagnosed with cancer.

I had ignored my health for nearly two decades because my family needed me to be there for them as a husband and father. But I failed them because I failed myself.

This may seem morbid, but I had to be alive and well for me to be the man I needed to be for them. But the path I followed at the time, littered with all the unhealthy decisions I made along the way, was the fast track to 300 lbs., 350 lbs., and beyond—or worse.

The thought of dying before Zach experienced milestone moments in his life—his first day of school, high school graduation, his wedding day, a family of his own—scared the life out of me.

As did the thought of being unable to take care of my family while Shelly focused on fighting a battle to save her life. But that can be reality when you lose control of your life, especially of your health and well-being, and you have felt powerless to change it for so long. I couldn't wait any longer to learn if that would be my reality. I had to change, or life sooner or later would take the choice out of my hands.

I don't recall how much money I paid to work with that coach on the way to losing seventy-five lbs. twelve years ago. You can't put a price on gaining the healthiest version of yourself and having the opportunity to hold onto it for dear life. If I were to crunch the financial numbers, though, the return on that pivotal investment exponentially exceeded whatever I paid. You wouldn't be reading this if I didn't bet on myself.

The proverbial snowball effect that has unfolded since then would have been an uphill battle if I had been too scared to say yes to that coach, if I had allowed the customary excuses that often ran through my mind convince me that the status quo was the way to go.

The momentum I have gained, like the confidence I have in myself, have led me down a life-altering path that revealed more about me and the man I have become than the weight I lost.

Losing weight was merely the vehicle to greater accomplishments that I never imagined then.

The husband I should be. The father I need to be. Health and fitness coach. Entrepreneur. Business owner. Published author. I'm as happy as I have ever been. How could I have imagined that?

Before I started my journey, I didn't believe in myself. I was destined to be unhealthy inside and out, unhappy with the man I had become, and unable to do anything to change it. As time passed, I began to notice physical change in my body and I realized I was doing what it took to be the healthiest version of myself.

I didn't look beyond the present. Fat melted away. Lean muscle grew. Getting out of bed in the morning was satisfying, not a struggle.

I was on track to my goal of being healthy. It's the goal for many of us whose health and fitness has gone from priority to convenience, and finally, an afterthought. We gauge progress by what we see in the mirror and wearing a pair of jeans we haven't fit into in years.

I focused each day on getting to the gym, doing my workout, and making good choices in the kitchen when cookies and chips and other goodies stared me in the face. I chose not to know what the future held. Too often in the past, looking to the future meant starting over again because the outcome was the same: a few weeks, maybe a month or two, of doing the work followed by completely falling off track due to poor choices and bad habits.

At the time, I was a married father of three sons, and well into a twenty-six-year career as a sports journalist. Until then, sports writing was both my passion and number one priority, because it was how I paid the bills and put a roof over our heads and food on the table. It consumed my life. I was so concerned about failing at my passion, so it always came first.

As my health deteriorated, my weight had ballooned to a high of 248.2 lbs. in my thirties. (I will always remember that number, down to the ounce, to remind myself of the depths I sank to so I would never return to that place again.) I looked and felt much older than I was. Meanwhile, life passed me by because I was merely existing within it and not living it to the fullest. Worse, my family suffered because of it. I was always working—at home, on the road, early in the day, late in the evening, all week long, and all weekend long as well—until the day that coach looked me in the eyes and, through her words, forced me to take control of my life. As I began to progress physically, the perspective on my life changed too.

If I made changes I once never thought possible, what was stopping me from pursuing goals that never used to be a part of my wildest dreams, much less ones I considered possible? I discovered my passion for sports journalism was merely the source of a paycheck, a way to take care of my family in the way I thought I was supposed to. What my family wanted was me at my best, at my happiest. Four months later, I became a certified personal trainer with an opportunity to share the many lessons I learned on my journey.

I'm different in so many ways now, possibly in more ways than I even realize. Now, as I help others change their lives and those of their families through health and fitness, they learn what I have learned: to allow the work they do in life to impact the goals they set in all aspects of their lives, personally and professionally.

Clients often hear me say, "If the goals you set don't make a certain set of cheeks pucker, you're not thinking big enough." As they achieve goals once considered unreachable, they learn anything is possible if they take the same approach to accomplish goals that change lives.

To be the best people we can be, for ourselves and those around us, we have to prioritize the most precious commodity we have: our health. For many of us, that's the most daunting challenge we will face in life, one that requires facing our biggest fears.

Mine was being a failure to my family. Zach is twelve years old now, and an avid student and athlete and all-around good kid. Shelly has been cancer free for eleven years, and an unwavering supporter of mine. She believes in the path I have chosen to follow, and the passion I have for helping others find their path to better health and fitness, and a way of life they have dreamed of but never pursued.

As for me, I'm a lucky man. Life could have unfolded far differently if I had continued down the path I followed for many years and continued to be believe the excuses that plagued my life.

Wasting all those years remains my biggest regret. I will take that regret to my grave. Still, that thought pushes me every day to help others avoid that same feeling.

So I ask you... *"Can you afford not to?"* You can't afford to allow control of your life to slip away. You desire to live a long, fulfilling life, but desire without action accomplishes nothing. It's time to take that first step, and I absolutely recommend hiring a health and fitness coach to guide you on your journey—a coach who understands the struggles we all face when we fail to prioritize our health and well-being for ourselves and our families.

Reach out to me at info@fernandesfit.com and let's take that step together, and the next and the next. Your goals will come into focus, and the life you want will grow very clear.

With the memory of shedding a life-changing seventy-five lbs. in his heart, Victor Fernandes made the choice to pursue passion over paychecks. He ended a twenty-six-year career in sports journalism in February 2019—at 47 years old—to help small business owners with families build the lives they covet, personally and professionally, by first taking control of their health and fitness. He loves seeing people create the best versions of themselves, in all facets of life, while serving as a leader by example for their families and generations to come... because he has seen what practicing what he preaches has done for him and his family.

CHAPTER TWO:
A Trip To The Gym—My Life's Biggest Catalyst

By Jerry Handley, M.S., M.S., CSCS, SCCC

Coach (\kohch\, noun).

1. *A passionate, dedicated individual who unlocks hidden potential and maximizes performance by believing, encouraging, and developing.*

I was a thirteen-year-old chubby kid—good at school, decent at baseball, and absolutely hooked at video games. Really no different than a lot of kids now, or a lot of kids in the '90s back then, and maybe not so different than you reading this book.

No one would have expected how my life would be changed by a simple invitation into a local YMCA weight room.

It started the day my best friend's mom got a family personal training package, and thinking her son could use some company to make it more enjoyable, she invited me along. For reasons I don't remember (probably just to hang out or be seen as cool by my friend), I accepted! Everyone—me included, honestly—thought I would be the first one to quit, since nothing in my past had indicated any interest in fitness. But something took hold…

All I did was give it an honest shot. I paid attention to the trainer. I worked hard at the exercises the trainer gave us. Even when my friend or his mom couldn't make it, I still got dropped off at the gym for my workout session. The workouts were activating a system in my personality I always had: achievement. Each exercise I could do better than the last time, I knew I had achieved improvement. It was a feeling that kept feeding me, and that fuel was enough to start a fire.

Coincidentally I also realized that while not many people may understand it, strength training was allowing my previous love of video games to come to life. Now when I would go home, I would build levels for my characters, but when I was at the gym, I would get to build up myself.

One simple "Yes" to the question, "Would you like to give a personal trainer a shot?" and the entire rest of my life had changed. Eventually I was no longer the chubby kid. I went from assuming I would be a doctor (which is what everyone in my family had said I would be from day one) to wanting to help others as a trainer before they needed medical care. I wanted to help people transform their bodies, for health or for performance.

I had begun lifting when I was thirteen, and it was at fifteen when I took the next step and got hooked on everything that could be achieved through exercise. For those first two years I had done the same program the personal trainer had given me. With no guidance after those first couple of months, I just kept doing the same thing… until I learned there could be more.

I went into a deep dive learning as much as I could—magazines, websites (that was 1998… there weren't many of those yet!), books, and I used myself as a guinea pig for what I learned.

I loved the variables: exercises, sets, reps, intensities, percentages, rest periods, intensity techniques, and more. I had gotten hooked on training science because I was a huge nerd, and all the variables that could be manipulated to create outcomes excited me. (I still am a huge nerd by the way, nerds never die.) The variables to me were like the ultimate puzzle or the greatest of applicable math equations. The act of training itself was like trying to create the greatest video game character possible, trying to max my stats and levels (I repeat, nerd).

There was more to the benefits from training, of course. While I mentioned being a chubby early teen, what I didn't mention is that I was the neighborhood Puerto Rican kid who had a mustache in middle school. In fact, I think it started coming in around fifth grade.

My self-esteem was amazing… amazingly low, that is. Chubby. Kid mustache. As I started to train, the self-esteem grew. Physically I was becoming stronger. When I started taking nutrition seriously, I became leaner. I became more confident not just outwardly, but inwardly as well from overcoming challenge after challenge. I was slowly realizing that fitness training is one of the greatest self-development tools in existence, and it's right there for all of us to grab and use starting any day we want. Including today.

Fast forward to when I graduated from high school. By then I knew I didn't want to treat sick people through medicine. I wanted to do something involving my passion of exercise. I discovered strength and conditioning as a freshman in college and decided that would be my future. What I hadn't learned yet was that training people to exercise was not the same as coaching. It was one of those days I'll never forget in February 2005, a freezing, snowy winter's morning in Morgantown, West Virginia, the day I really learned about being a "coach."

At twenty-one I was the youngest coach on the Strength & Conditioning staff at West Virginia University. The athletes were my age and some even had a year or two on me. At that time, everything about coaching had been going smoothly, but almost TOO smoothly…

Everything I had done was focused on learning more about training science and wanting to train others. When asked questions, I would give highly scientific answers that made almost no sense to the listener. I knew it meant I would be successful at training others, particularly athletes; after all, I knew they would be the hardest-working, most committed trainees on the planet! And that my friends… is where I was dead wrong.

As soon as I landed my first official position as a Strength Coach, I learned college athletes were just like anyone else. They had demanding schedules, talent, and skills, and had worked hard to become a college athlete, but that didn't automatically mean they were any more driven than you or me.

Not all college athletes were motivated. Not all of them were dreaming of the next level. Not all of them were even in shape! And at 5:30 a.m. in the middle of winter… ALL OF THEM were tired!

It was the type of pre-dawn workout with one express purpose: to break people. This wasn't the strength staff's doing, the football coaches designed these team workouts. We strength coaches were just the ones who made the wheels turn while the sports coaches "graded" the players on effort, lazy plays, and mistakes. They looked for reasons to yell and give mistake checkmarks; that was their whole plan that far from the season, wanting to build toughness and grit in their team. (I am neither supporting nor condemning this plan, just reporting the facts!)

I was coaching an agility station, running the rotating groups of players through different combinations of changes in direction. The guys were NOT doing well with lots of mistakes, incorrect running patterns, and sloppy and slow movements. The usual coaching cues to do the right things just weren't working. Meanwhile, the sports coaches were heating up everywhere, and you could tell there was a crazy energy in the facility. The head coach started screaming at every station he stopped, and athletes just began to fall apart.

Then something inside me clicked. It was no longer about strictly coaching movement and pointing out corrections to be made. This wasn't just another day of creating patterns from a textbook on a field around cones.

Coaching is about LEADING PEOPLE. The tone in my voice changed and became stronger, louder, and more motivating. It was about pushing each individual to do their best, not just to try harder. As each player realized I was coaching FOR THEM, the intensity picked up, and so did the attention to detail. Suddenly the group at my station was killing it!

After a few minutes the head coach finally made his way over to my station. He watched for several minutes, only speaking a handful of times, and when he did speak, it was commending the individuals for their effort, or reminding them to listen to me. He walked away and the atmosphere in the rest of the facility changed because his energy had changed.

That day, I felt a different sense of what I could do by directing my energy into training others. My boss said at a staff meeting later that it had been my efforts that saved the day from the head coach's wrath. As a young strength coach, that positive criticism made a lifelong impact and taught me one of the most valuable lessons I keep in mind almost two decades later: With exercise as my tool, it is within my power to guide others to greatness through service. And that is my purpose.

Jerry "The East Coast Viking" Handley found his true passion when opening Viking Performance Training LLC in 2014, a passion centered around helping everyone achieve fitness and athletic goals while building confidence, particularly school-aged clients. Handley spent over a decade as a championship strength coach and professor at West Virginia University before opening VPT and has trained Olympic medalists, World Champions, NBA and MLB draft picks, All-Americans, and other professional athletes, as well as helped hundreds of athletes earn college scholarships. What fuels him the most? Helping people of all ages train to become their best self.

Interested in a personalized training program that will help you reach your specific goals of feeling more confident and stronger at the same time? Contact Jerry through any of the following:

Email: vikingperformancetraining@gmail.com
Website: www.vikingperformancetraining.com

LinkedIn: https://www.linkedin.com/in/jerry-handley-14a6b5141
Facebook:
https://www.facebook.com/VikingPerformanceTraining
Instagram self: https://www.instagram.com/realjerryhandley/
Instagram gym:
https://www.instagram.com/therealvikingperformance/

CHAPTER THREE:
A Lifechanging Journey

By Jessica Ledbetter

It was nearing the end of 2020 and I had no hope left. As I sat at home in isolation with my three kids, I looked around and really absorbed how sad my life was. The house was a wreck. Dishes filled the sink, the kids' toys and clothes were strewn through the place. I wanted to clean but I just couldn't get myself up to take care of anything. My mental health was at its lowest and I had been diagnosed with postpartum depression. It didn't help that we had been quarantining and my husband worked out of town. I had no help and no support system. My baby was nearing three months old, and her sisters were only four and five years old. There was constant crying, fighting, and chaos in my house, and I found myself responding poorly. I felt like an awful mother. It was time to take a hard look in the mirror and make some changes, if not for me… for my children.

I grew up in a very toxic environment. At the age of five I witnessed my mother go into labor at home, place my newborn brother into a garbage bag, and hide it under her bed. She hemorrhaged shortly after and passed away that night. My father abandoned me and turned to alcohol. I grew up moving between family members and dealing with a lot of abuse. I had no idea how to be a mom, no clue what moms do. All I ever knew was that I didn't want my children to ever feel a quarter of the pain I endured growing up. I started to recognize that this depression was making me be an awful person. I would snap and get upset over the stupidest things. My patience was thin, and I felt like the girls might honestly be better off without me. I didn't know what to do or how to beat it without medicating myself, so I turned to Google and started researching ways to combat depression on my own naturally. Little did I know, this was the first step into a fitness journey that would forever change me for the better.

I read that working out daily and eating more nutritiously would help me feel better, so I started my lifechanging journey that day. I had no idea where to begin. Quite frankly, I had never worked out before. I weighed 246 lbs. and grew up eating mostly ramen and Hot Pockets. My knowledge was zero when it came to eating healthy. Google became my best friend as I started looking up healthy recipes and workouts I could do from home. I only worked out for five minutes that first day, but it was a start.

Working out was HARD. I felt like I was dying after doing a warm-up, but I stayed consistent. I didn't feel better immediately, and honestly, I felt like it was stupid. I was questioning if working out was worth it at all. The only thing I had gained from it so far was soreness. A friend of mine suggested that I develop a routine listening to something motivational as soon as I woke up every day. I thought that was stupid too, but I did it anyway. Mindset is such an important skill to work on, especially when it comes to your fitness. Developing personally will help you push through even when you feel less than motivated.

After a few weeks of consistency, I began to feel like I was climbing out of my depressed state. I started to look forward to my workouts, and I even ordered some resistance bands and dumbbells. My mental state was slowly changing, and I started to feel like a fighter instead of someone who was willing to give up on it all. A month passed and I no longer felt suicidal, plus I lost almost eight lbs.! I learned quickly in my journey that consistency was key to successfully reaching my goals. Being consistent on the days you feel like crap, the days you're overwhelmed and overstimulated, and even the days you're just plain busy and short on time, is how you create a real lifestyle change.

I couldn't have done any of this without my friend Eric King encouraging me. Eric came in like a wrecking ball, breaking down the walls I had built around myself, calling my phone regularly with encouragement and advice that really helped me continue pushing forward. I had met Eric a few years prior when I worked in a convenience store. He was a regular customer that always put a smile on my face when he came in to buy a newspaper.

Eric was older and wiser than me, and he was also a pastor and personal trainer. He stepped into my life and became the positive parent-type figure that I had never had before. After a few months of my working out and eating right, Eric mentioned to me that I should become a trainer. I had become very passionate and almost addicted to progress, but I laughed at him that day. I had never imagined that I could have a future career in the fitness industry. I continued to spend my time focusing on my health and pushing myself to become a little better each day.

By the time March 2021 rolled around, I felt like a new person. I had lost forty lbs., stayed consistent with my meal plan, and managed to smile again. My older girls were registered to play tee-ball for the first time, and I was so excited to see them play. Right before the season began, the director let me know that if they didn't have a volunteer to coach that there would be no tee-ball that year. I really wanted my children to have the opportunity to play but I was in no position to coach them. I played softball one year when I was nine, but I really just picked flowers in the outfield...

The thought of volunteering to coach kept nagging me and the motivational videos I had been listening to every morning had really started to do work on my mindset. My inner self reflected on doing uncomfortable things to push myself to new limits. I decided that coaching the kids would challenge me and could be my next step to getting out of the house and back into the world. How hard could it be?

Oh, my goodness! Coaching a team of kids between the ages of five and seven is not for the weak. With my husband working out of town most of the time and my baby was still breastfeeding, my best option was to coach with her strapped to my chest in an infant carrier. We were a sight to see and thank God I had built up my strength because my child seemed to get heavier each day. Although it was hard, being outside and watching those kids improve throughout the season really helped me continue to feel better, and even hopeful, for the future.

It was at the end of the season when I reflected on the growth of the team and began to really recognize and appreciate the growth in myself. I had lost fifty-seven lbs. at this point and began to realize that I found my passion. I followed Eric's advice and started to take the steps I needed to become a personal trainer. My own lifestyle changes and progress throughout my fitness journey almost seemed unreal, like it was too good to be true.

I still had a way to go before my body was in its best shape, but this had been a major year of growth for me, and I was on fire with motivation. By the time I completed my certification, I had lost eighty lbs. and that old, depressed mindset was in the rearview mirror. I kept pushing myself to do the uncomfortable, and in 2022, I ran my first marathon and competed in a transformation body building show.

The house is no longer a wreck, and my life isn't sad anymore. My children are running through the place with smiles on their faces, my patience has returned, and I'm living a life I never thought was possible. Fitness is more than just working out. Fitness is making time to take care of your mindset and nutrition as well. Focusing on my overall fitness shifted my future and changed my life. Who knows where I would be now if I didn't take that hard look in the mirror a few years ago?

As I look around and absorb the life I have today, I'm filled with gratitude and joy for the lessons I learned along the way. Be consistent with not only your workouts and eating habits, but with your personal development as well. Always push yourself to do the uncomfortable things, and you won't regret the growth that's connected to it. Don't be afraid to get out of your own way.

Do research and take good advice; there's always something we can learn. The most important thing I learned was to love myself at all stages of the journey and make a habit of working on my personal development. We all too often are our own worst critics, but it's a game changer when you start to focus on what your body can do instead of hating it for what it's not doing.

If you struggle with depression and obesity, I challenge you to take that long hard look in the mirror like I did. Make a change and start it today. We have one life. Why waste it not becoming the best version of yourself?

If I can change my life, so can you. Send an email to jessicaledbetter95@icloud.com and mention this book for a free fitness consult.

I would love to help you shift your path.

Jessica Ledbetter is married to her best friend Adam and is a mother to three daughters. She's transformed her life through fitness and is passionate about helping others who suffer with depression and obesity establish healthy lifestyle changes of their own. Jessica is a Certified Personal Trainer, Nutritionist, and a Weight Management Specialist. She believes in operating with the core values of gratitude, respect, integrity, and transparency. You can connect best with Jessica on Facebook https://www.facebook.com/jessica.davis.7965 *or Instagram @blestjessfitness*

CHAPTER FOUR:
A Fitness Professional Fighting An Uphill Battle

By Josh Riggs

My story begins similarly to many others, as a chubby kid who grew up in the midst of diet culture in the mid '90s and early 2000s. Being overweight going into middle school is less than ideal and anyone who has experienced that can vouch. It ultimately led me down a miserable path of body dysmorphia for the next fifteen years. Growing up in poverty, there weren't exactly the best nutritional options available, nor did I have much of an understanding of nutrition at the time. What I did know was what societal, medical, and media influence suggested to lose weight was to eat less. So, I started there.

By this time, I'd already fallen victim to anorexia, unbeknownst to me at the time so I'll paint the scene for you:

It's 5 a.m. and I have three hours to myself before I have to get ready for class at Chauncey Rose Middle School. I wake up, roll out of bed, and feel exhausted, but this is a norm for me. I hop on the scale and weigh in at 112 lbs. at 5'11". "Dang! I still have two lbs. to lose." I weigh out my cereal to exactly a half-portion size and eat it as slowly as I can. The whole time dreading the fact that I would have to go to school where people will make fun of me for being so skinny. I never understood why they said that because when I looked in the mirror, I still saw nothing but the chubby boy I once was. I finish my breakfast, still hungry, but such is life as I knew it. I spend the rest of the day thinking about my next meal of a banana and some peanut butter before cross country practice. After a solid four miles of running, I finally got to go back to bed to start it all over again.

This was my life day in and day out. Everyone was either worried about me or making fun of me, but I did not care. All that mattered to me was not being fat. I didn't know it then, but I had severe anorexia. In fact, I really had no idea what that even was until I got to high school. I had a PE teacher who was almost at bodybuilder status. He was massive, like the Dragon Ball Z characters (anime that I watched regularly) that I thought looked so cool. I told him I wanted to look like that and explained what I was doing to get there. Luckily for me, he was nice enough to teach me what I was doing wrong.

Mr. Ellis spent the next two years doing what no other therapist, school bully, or even my own grandparents could do. He changed my mindset on how I looked and taught me what I needed to do to get to where I wanted to be. He would work out with me every day after school and had me tell him how much I was eating. He would make small changes. An extra egg here, some chicken there, until before long, I was slowly starting to feel better and look better. He told me to throw my scale away (which, to this day, was one of the harder things I've had to do) and had me cover up every mirror I could. Before long, I fell in love with the new routine: eat, work out, eat more. It was great!

By the time I graduated, I was up to 140 lbs. I was still super lean but had far more muscle. I wanted to build on what Mr. Ellis had taught me and learn everything I could about the human body. I took every free course I could and even got my CPT from NASM (National Academy of Sports Medicine). I found a new purpose: to try and get as big as I could and help as many people avoid what I went through as possible.

I kept upping my calories and lifting harder and harder, following every tip I learned along the way. Eventually, friends and family began seeking me out for advice and help toward their own goals so naturally I took a step toward training people to better themselves. Before long they were getting amazing results as well. In fact, they were getting better results than I was. This stumped me and I could not figure why it seemed like it took far more effort for me than for them. I was eating as much as I could every day (which at the time was about 3,000 calories) but was going nowhere. Even though everyone else I was training was blowing up with muscle! I hit a plateau.

I had my hormones checked and found out that I had severely low testosterone. I mean, really really low! It explained all kinds of things, including why my voice never changed. The doctor suggested that I begin TRT (synthetic testosterone) and told me I would never be able to achieve anything if I didn't. Something about that did not sit well with me so I went out of my way to prove him wrong.

I spent the next five years eating 5,000-plus calories every day, lifting harder than ever. I worked harder than anyone I knew. I was always exhausted, always sick of eating, and hated every second of it. However, I never gave up. After five years I managed to put on fifteen lbs. of muscle. It was slow and it was hard but I was winning. Then I hit a huge roadblock: I got dumped.

My girlfriend of eight years called it off abruptly and it sent me down a dark path. This person, who had experienced a significant part of my journey with me, who had been supportive of my goals despite not having much interest in fitness herself, more or less just up and left. I quickly lost fifteen lbs. in two months—the fifteen lbs. that took me five years to gain! I felt defeated and alone. Not long after, however, there came a person that kept showing up during this time. Tori. Interestingly, she actually began as a client of mine. I know, how cliché. As unconventional as it was and can typically be deemed as unprofessional, there was a strong connection between us that otherwise saved me from myself.

Tori went out her way to check on me post break-up and got me up and moving. She invited me to go on walks with her and her dog. She went with me on camping trips and other fun adventures. She helped me get back into the routine that I had thrown out the window and encouraged me to enjoy life for the first time. Needless to say, I ended up falling for her and I fired her as my client so that we could enjoy life together more conventionally.

It was not long before she moved in, and being the not-so-great cook that I am, she started cooking for us instead. She made eating far less of a chore and getting that 5,000 calories in was so much easier. At some point, she found out about my low testosterone issue and strongly encouraged me to get it fixed for more reasons than just gym gains. Low testosterone affects so many components in a man's ability to function on a daily basis that I hadn't really put much thought in before. I didn't sleep well, I was constantly exhausted and irritable, I was always hungry, etc. So finally, I took a leap of faith, started TRT, and got my levels up in the healthy range. I was, however, concerned that in balancing my hormones synthetically, people would begin to discredit the work I had put in and not be as impressed with my capabilities. What I learned was that I was the only one trying to discredit my work and abilities as it related to my hormones.

I went back to my same lifting routine but this time what had taken me five years only took six to eight months and on significantly fewer calories, right around 3,000 to 3,500. I was able to incorporate more balance into my life and accept that I did not need to eat in such a detrimentally strict manner to accomplish my goals. I was able to find food freedom.

I managed to put on more lean muscle and hold onto it more effectively than ever. I was recovering from workouts more efficiently; my body was finally working with me rather than against me. I so badly wanted to prove that doctor wrong that I made myself so miserable for so long, I had a hard time imagining anything different. I was able to accomplish far more than I should have been able to with such low testosterone levels, but I realized I did not have to compromise my wellness at the expense of an emotionally unhelpful medical professional.

My mindset has drastically changed when it comes to health and fitness over the last year or so. I no longer feel as though everything is an uphill battle, and at long last feel like I can reach my fitness goals the same way I help others reach theirs.

Josh Riggs have been in the fitness industry for six years. During that time, he has gone from part-time trainer to owning and operating multiple gym locations. He currently owns West Indy Barbell and Dedicated Health along with his partners. He has helped countless people reach their fitness goals, and is on a mission to help communities live better lives through fitness, education, and support.

CHAPTER FIVE:
Building A Solid Foundation

By Marilyn Hoyt

Our journey shapes us for our purposes in life. Mine has been interesting—from a prissy drill team girl, a hardcore Army woman, to a cancer survivor, and business owner. Life throws us many lessons to shape us to become a better version of ourselves.

I grew up as an only child who would get bored and do a few little workouts to entertain myself. In high school, I tried out for the drill team (dance team), and that became my passion and source of fun during those years. I got drill team scholarships to go to college, but during my senior year, I moved out of my parents' house and ended up losing the scholarships.

After graduating from high school, I had a front desk position and would complete all my work by lunch time. I was bored and lost with life. Prissy little me decided to walk into an Army office and ask the recruiter if I had to cut my hair to join.

Vain? Maybe.

But he said no and we talked. I took all of the Army information and went to my friend's house. My friends looked at me in disbelief that I would even consider joining, and that pushed me to want to do it more! So, prissy little me did!

I arrived at Ft. Leonard Wood, Missouri, with drill sergeants yelling and ordering us around. It was pure chaos. I weighed barely 100 lbs. with no muscle but with a bull-headed mind. We had to carry a load on our back that weighed as much as I did and it was wearing out my tiny body. We ran all day every day and I just couldn't catch my breath. I felt like my lungs were collapsing. I remember saying, I can't breathe, and the drill sergeant made a point to remind me if you are talking, you are breathing. Little did I know the boots that were made for men and the weight on my back would cause a setback for me.

When you are in training to be a soldier of the U.S. Army, you don't want to look or feel weak. To go to the clinic, called sick call, was a disgrace. My ankles were strained and running or walking caused so much pain for me. One of my drill sergeants noticed my limp. He yelled out, "Private!! Take your boot off." I was busted. Dang it!! I sat down and had to pry my boot off my foot. The drill sergeant ordered me to go to sick call. Doctors examined me and diagnosed stress fractures in both ankles, plus my arches had fallen due to having to carry double my weight around. I came back on crutches and my spirit broken and pride gone. I was worried.

I needed to practice running for my final test and didn't want to redo two months of basic training.

I was bull headed and determined, so I was off of crutches in two weeks. I had two more weeks to practice a run I had barely passed. I remember that on the testing day it was 32 degrees outside. I took off all my cover-ups and figured I would run faster since I was cold. It worked!!! I passed my run and graduated basic training. In my mind I knew I would need to put in the work to get better on running. I got to my first duty station and ran at least four days a week. I ended up maxing my Physical Fitness Test and getting my fitness patch.

Running got easier and I found myself motivating other soldiers. I became a non-commissioned officer E-5, and since I was good in fitness, my first sergeant put me in charge of the soldiers having issues passing the physical fitness test. I found a passion in helping others build stamina and strength, reminding each soldier that it was our job to take care of our bodies and to be fit soldiers. I served six years and then came back to the civilian world with a soldier mentality.

I joined an all-women gym and worked out for about two hours a day while my boys stayed in the childcare. Other members started to ask me questions about different equipment and I was excited to teach them how to use the equipment. The instructors for the group workouts loved my energy and enthusiasm in their workouts. A few instructors asked me to become certified but I didn't believe I could actually be in front and lead a workout.

After a year, an instructor approached me again, and this time added they would sponsor me to get certified in Turbo Kick. I was shocked and honored they believed in me so much they would sponsor me. I got the certification and started working in the gym doing sales and miscellaneous things. The front desk had a call come in at 8 a.m. from the 9 a.m. group workout instructor letting them know she wouldn't be able to make it in. They turned to me and asked if I could fill in. Eeeekkkk!!

Are you serious?!? I said okay, got some yellow Post-It notes, and wrote out a total body workout. I got in front of the gym members and seriously fell in love. I was conducting a group workout with ease and it was tough. I was a drill sergeant at a female gym. I ended up taking over the 9 a.m. body blaster workout and was nicknamed Sgt. Body Killer.

As I was working at the all-women gym, I met Annette, who was passionate about helping others get fit. Her training style was opposite from mine. She and I decided to venture out and start boot camps and in-home personal training. She was the sweet trainer and I was the tough one. She and I decided to leave the all-women gym and go somewhere else while we worked on our new business.

We went back and forth with names but one stuck. Rock. Why? Rock is a strong foundation. God is our foundation.

We want our clients to establish a good solid foundation in their life to create healthy habits.

Rock Fitness it is! Let's do this!

Marketing at schools, churches, and businesses, Annette and I had a good partnership and friendship. We were busy and life was good. No weekends or late nights, which was perfect for me since I just became a single mom of two boys ages seven and four. We were impacting lives. I was the tough trainer making everyone do toe pushups and pushing hard. It doesn't matter how you feel you have to be tough. Get your body fit and able. We will get results. I was Sgt. Body Killer. A trainer with an Army soldier attitude. After almost a year of rocking Rock Fitness, my health was attacked at the end of 2010.

I was a single mom and a new business owner, and I was about to be taken down again—but this time harder. I am known as a tough woman who doesn't allow things to get to her—a woman who keeps it all together—but this challenge would test me even more than ever.

I was getting up at 5 a.m. to do early morning group workouts and running kids to school. I was extremely exhausted and would have to nap all the time. I figured it was due to lack of sleep. I started to zone into my nutrition because I had a sweet tooth and wanted to practice what I was teaching my clients. Plus, I wanted to be healthy on the inside and out. I was still tired and knew something was off. I went in to get a check-up and they told me there was a strong chance I had cancer but it could be removed with surgery, and as long as it wasn't in my lymph nodes, I would be fine.

I was in complete shock. How does a healthy and fit person get hit with this? I resolved to do what I needed to do and I would be fine. Everyone doesn't need to know. It's no one's business and I don't want to hear all the "I'm so sorrys" from people. Plus, I have a business to grow and boys to raise. Let's get this surgery done so I can get moving!

Surgery was done and they had scrapped some lymph nodes. I would get the results during the holidays. My doctor called me into her office on December 26. She told me she wanted me to have a good Christmas but my lymph nodes had come back with cancer and I would need to undergo chemotherapy and radiation. I had gone to this appointment alone and the rest of the information she told me was only mumbles to me.

How did this happen to me? What about my boys? They were young. I had to fight. I had to maintain my composure. I had to be strong. Rock Fitness had to take a back seat. My cancer was invasive since it was in my lymphatic system. I was faced with needed a full hysterectomy (which means also hormone treatment) and a strong possibility of radiation. I had to go to Dallas to see the oncologist and he would take x-rays of my lungs to make sure it hadn't spread that far.

My emotions were up and down. I cried a lot. I'm not an emotional person who cries easily, so I cried a lot for myself!

Believers said to me that when you start following Christ and living the way He calls us to live, we are attacked.

I had a wide range of emotions, but no matter what my emotions were screaming I knew the TRUTH! I knew and believed God was healing me and teaching me. I can praise Him for all and cast ALL my anxiety on HIM because HE cares for ME! I'm a fighter when I HAVE to be—plus I'm a little hard headed. I carried my cross and was ready to kick some ASS along with my prayer warriors.

I clung to a favorite Bible verse, 2 Corinthians 4:8-9. We are hard pressed on every side, BUT NOT CRUSHED, perplexed, BUT NOT IN DESPAIR, persecuted, but NOT ABANDONED. struck down, BUT NOT DESTROYED!

We are not promised a life of ease and comfort. We are not promised escape, rescue, tearless, pain-free living. We are guaranteed quite the opposite. We are promised, beyond the shadow of a doubt, God's presence, peace, joy—His very self through it all.

We are promised the heavy will become light when weighed against eternity. That is the promise I clasped onto for dear life. The promise that when everything feels as if it is crashing around you, that you will not survive, it is so very dark and more than you can take, you will be held—Held in the very palm of the Heavenly Father's hand. This is what I believed.

I had clients starting at 8 a.m. One of my clients had been praying for me and sent me a text after I got my bad results. She didn't know the outcome because I didn't tell her but she asked me if I got good news. I told her no, but it was time to work out. I gave her my details and told her negative thoughts had crossed my mind and I was trying to drown those out with God's truth.

She said to me, Isaiah 26:3, *You will keep in perfect peace those whose minds are steadfast, because they trust in you.*

She reminded me God is has this covered and I will have an awesome testimony. God used her to encourage me. My client inspired me and filled me with truth. After seeing my clients, I went on the treadmill to run off some frustration.

Listening to my music, zoning out, I could feel my tears filling my eyes and my adrenaline taking off, so I made my music louder and picked up my pace. I got off and ran the stairs. The main trainer manager was there and asked me if I was okay or if I needed anything. Then he informed me I could take a medical leave of absence and still keep my job. I didn't trust him. I then went to my car, put my sunglasses on, and cried for a little bit. I had four lymph nodes positive for cancer and would have to go through chemotherapy and radiation for eight weeks.

I started to think about spiritual growth. I told God I WANT TO TRUST HIM WITH ALL OF MY LIFE, I want to live with purpose, and to use me for all HIS glory. I told him I'm not ready to go home yet. I'm ready to fight, I'm ready to be God's soldier. I'm ready for him to train me for GREATNESS for HIM!

I'm amazed at how God can give this amazing peace in your heart even when you're scared. The people He puts in our lives to help us through our journeys. I'm running a marathon and I promise you I will finish strong because God is with me!

I've been struck down, but you know what? I'm not destroyed! The Lord is transforming me for greatness. This world tells us what we should do, tolerate, accept and or believe.

Do not conform any longer to the pattern of this world, but be transformed by the renewing of your mind. Then you will be able to test and approve what God's will is—his good, pleasing and perfect will!

—Romans 12:2

I continued to work out and train the few clients I had at the gym. Very few and selective people knew what was going on with me: my boss at the gym, my clients, friends and family who I knew would pray for me, and my kids' teachers.

Chemotherapy and radiation were easy at first. I drank a lot of water, read, journaled, and prayed for hours a day. Leaning on the Lord was the way I decided to fight my battle.

At the end of treatments, things caught up with me. My body was worn out, physically and mentally. I had three more treatments to go. I was going to work right after my treatments. I ended up with fever and dizziness. Lab work results indicated an infection. The doctor put me on antibiotics, and I stayed on the couch the whole day and night. I couldn't move and it hurt to walk. My sweet boys tried to get me to eat and be self-sufficient. It hurt I couldn't be the mom they needed me to be.

The next day they went to school and I couldn't get up to walk, I was in so much pain. I screamed. I couldn't handle it anymore, so I called 911. All I remember was yelling in pain. It was a very low point for me. I then got admitted to the hospital due to a low blood count, bladder infection, and a sack of fluid that was lying on my sciatic nerve which hindered my ability to walk. All I kept hearing was I was young and healthy and I would be okay.

Young?? Healthy?? Why the heck am I here??

Day after day went on as I lay on the hospital bed drugged up. Not able to be a mom or able to work. The blood transfusion was something I would never in my life thought I would have to go through. But this was not my plan—it's God's!

On the second night I told my Heavenly Father I had ENOUGH. I can't anymore. I JUST CAN'T. I WANT MY LIFE BACK. I could barely hold my eyes open to text. My

Heavenly Father held me in HIS arms. He continued to love me. He felt my pain and taught me to rest. It was the end of this adventure. God wired me for greatness, he made me stubborn, strong, independent. He had to break me—break me completely for complete healing. He had to break me to be dependent on HIM, strong with the HOLY SPIRIT. Taught me to be BOLD for Him! My Heavenly Father sent me little encouragement throughout my life. Many have come from Rock Fitness.

God slapped me across the face and taught me through cancer the importance of progressions. Your mind can tell you that you can do something but your body just can't. I had to rehab my leg. I limped for a long time. It gave me great respect for people's bodies. Understanding there are steps to get to the goal and results. That takes consistency and time.

I learned patience and empathy for my clients due to my recovery. I learned about hormones and the huge role they play in our weight loss, muscle building, and energy. I had to start to rebuild Rock Fitness and was thankful for clients who looked out for me at the gym.

Cancer is an uphill battle. It affects you emotionally, physically, mentally, spiritually, your family, finances, and everyday life. Everyone goes through something in their lives that is like cancer. You have to push forward and keep going. Life doesn't stop for the problems. Through God we can do all things. He is the one who provides the strength to move on when I can't anymore.

It was time to rebuild Rock Fitness. The clients I had at the gym where I was working saw how I was mistreated during this time and encouraged me to quit and work on Rock Fitness full time. I was nervous, but I did it.

Boy did it grow! Due to the trials I went through, I was a more attentive and understanding trainer—meaning it's not just about programming a good workout program, but knowing where this person is coming from, not just physically but mentally. Learning personalities and adapting to it. My boot camps in the park became more and I started to do mobile personal training. After five years, we moved to Farmersville, Texas.

The move made things harder for my business. I was newly married and now had three boys to transport. I had to arrange Rock Fitness boot camps and training around school activities and sporting activities. I was driving around way too much. I decided to build Rock Fitness out in Farmersville and started doing a boot camp at my youngest boy's school. I introduced myself to a local for-women-only Nautilus equipment gym, which was located in downtown Farmersville. I told them I would do a group workout for them for a few months.

A year later, the owner called me and asked if I wanted to take over the lease! I thought, no way! I can't handle the overhead and I don't like Nautilus equipment. I ended up taking it and Rock Fitness had its first location!

We were now in downtown Farmersville. I needed to develop a new business plan to attract more people. I decided to find a yoga instructor and other instructors to create a group workout fitness center. It was really nice to be out of the bad weather conditions, but I wanted to have more scheduled workouts for the community. I had an energetic Zumba instructor and filled our yoga spot. Later on, I had a friend who came on board who is yoga certified. Rock Fitness finally had a steady group fitness flow and we were growing!

Then 2020 happened. My lease was up after three years and all gyms had mandatory shutdowns. I went back into my garage and continued training clients. A few weeks later, I got a Facebook message from the only full gym owner in town, asking how I was holding up due to the shutdowns. We knew each other and they had checked out Rock Fitness. I let them know I was no longer downtown and back in my garage. They asked me to take over their facility and make it Rock Fitness. I immediately said no. They encouraged me and told me how I was really good at advertising for Rock Fitness and I could really grow if I took over. I took a deep breath, exhaled, and said, "Okay."

In June 2020, Rock Fitness moved into a 2,400 square foot gym, offering group workouts, personal training, and is now a 24/7 access full gym. Rock Fitness has truly been blessed. We've had so many people help grow it, make it successful, and make improvements along the way. I look forward to seeing Rock Fitness become more successful in the future as I work on becoming a wiser business woman.

Are you ready to build a solid foundation and live a life with quality and purpose?

Then it's time to join the Rock Fitness Tribe!

Click this link for your free consultation https://rockfitnesscamp.com/memberships

Marilyn is a disabled Army Veteran. In 2009 She became a turbo kick certified instructor, got her National Academy of Sports Medicine personal training certification, and taught weight resistance and cardio classes. In 2010, Marilyn teamed up with Annette Browning to start Rock Fitness Camp and became a part-time trainer at a big chain b8ix gym in Rowlett.

Shortly after, Marilyn was diagnosed with cancer and underwent chemotherapy and radiation treatments. She continued to train others and do as much as she could. During this time, Marilyn says God taught her so much about His love and how to trust Him with everything. Doctors also raved about her being physically healthy and how her fitness level contributed significantly to her recovery from cancer. God has healed her and she trains others with a purpose.

In 2016, she became a MoveMore Fitness Expert and also Certified in Calisthenics through Dragon Door. Marilyn's training style is motivating and encouraging. She will push

you when you are slacking and remind you why you are doing this, but she will also slow down those hardcore people who hurt themselves and need to rehabilitate. Fitness is important to battle life—physically & mentally!

CHAPTER SIX:
Four Critical Steps to Getting and Staying In Great Shape

By Marc Zalmanoff

I don't have a "fitness journey" story. I didn't lose a bunch of weight and inadvertently find my way into coaching.

My career began due to my inability to understand organic chemistry in college and a plethora of science credits I did not want to waste. This led to a bachelor's degree in kinesiology, which turned into becoming a personal trainer after graduating from the University of North Texas in 2002.

Fast forward 21 years later, and being a fitness professional has not only been part of my life throughout that entire time, but part of my identity as well. I found a passion serving people through exercise and discovered it's so much more than that. As coaches, we have the ability to truly effect lives on a deep level. Sure, we help people lose weight and eat better, but we also help boost self-esteem, regain confidence, walk a little taller, speak with more confidence, and feel better from the inside out.

Health and fitness, as I've seen it, is a microcosm of how someone lives their life. Show me a fit person and I'll show you someone who is typically successful (however you want to define success) in other areas of life.

Having coached more people than I can account for, I've certainly seen some commonalities amongst those who find long term success in getting and staying in great physical condition. I believe if you're willing to adopt these four tenets of health and wellness, you will find the same success in your journey.

Make a Decision

Every change we make in life begins with a decision. While it seems simple enough, this is often the hardest part of the process. It's no secret that regular exercise and proper nutrition benefit your overall health and quality of life. So, if we know that, why do so few people pursue it?

Because it's hard.

And as soon as we decide we've had enough of being fat, and overweight, and getting out of breath walking up the stairs, and complaining of how our back hurts, and feeling lethargic all the time, etc., then we must take action.

Every client I've ever coached who was successful had reached a point in their health where they knew something had to change. For some it was facing the option of back surgery or weight loss. For others it was becoming a parent or grandparent and realizing they wouldn't be able to play with a child because they were so out of shape. Many simply got tired of avoiding the person staring back at them in the mirror.

Regardless of the prompt, a decision was made that was followed by action. But without the decision itself, nothing would ever change. Be willing to boldly decide you deserve better and make a choice to change.

Be Consistent

I have a client who's been coaching with me since July 2008. In case you don't realize, that's a long time to be enrolled in any type of coaching program, much less one you have to physically show up for multiple times a week.

My man Dale has degenerative discs in his low back, which is not something you can fix. However, you can strengthen all the muscles that support your lower back, your midsection, your legs, and your upper back, which all contribute to the discs themselves not being as stressed.

Dale knew when we started working together that he was in it for the long haul. There would be days he could barely walk upright and he knew it would take time to correct. So, he made a commitment to come to the gym at least three days a week.

Week after week, month after month, year after year, Dale kept showing up. He swore he would never run, then he found himself doing 5Ks. His "bad back" then carried him through various obstacle course races, including a fifteen-mile Warrior Dash that we completed together. Combine that with ten Tough Mudders, deadlifts over 400 lbs., pullups for days, and generally being a guinea pig for whatever shenanigans I come up with in the gym, and I'd say his consistency has paid off tremendously.

One of the biggest mistakes people make when starting a new exercise program is not allowing their body to properly adapt. When you show up on day one, you're going to be sore. But if you wait until the soreness subsides before you show up again, you're going to be equally as sore. However, if you get a consistent schedule and stay committed to it, that soreness will dissipate faster, and your body will adapt to the new stimulus with greater ease.

Commit to consistency.

Put Things on the Calendar

Working out for health reasons is great. I believe it should be the overall purpose of regular physical activity. In a society of flashy things and short attention spans, I have discovered people can often get bored even with the most effective programs. One thing that has helped me personally, and helped many of my clients over the years, is putting something on the calendar that requires you to be better.

For example, I started doing Tough Mudders back in 2013. I had no idea what I was getting myself into and none of my clients wanted to do them with me. So I did it, had a blast, and came back super excited to tell the tale! My excitement paid off and the following spring I had a handful of clients join me for the next one. For a couple of months prior to the event, we trained a little differently and I noticed those who signed up were super consistent, more so than usual.

Hmmm, we were onto something. We wanted to feel prepared. We wanted to stay injury free. We wanted to get on the course and have fun, not feel like we'd gotten the crap kicked out of us!

Over the years I've found that by having periodic events on the calendar—Tough Mudders, 5Ks, 10Ks, half marathons, Strongman Competitions—it keeps us training on the days we don't feel like it. It pushes us out of our comfort zone to demand more of our bodies. It allows us to put our fitness to the test and do more than just "lift weights and do cardio."

I encourage you to try new things to see what you enjoy, then always keep something on the calendar to keep you striving for more.

Adopt a "Fit" Mindset

Have you ever met someone who lost a bunch of weight, only to gain it back? Or perhaps you know someone who was working out religiously, then all of sudden they're back to zero activity? We all know people who have seemingly struggled their entire life with trying to get in shape, to no avail. I firmly believe the difference in people who get and stay fit for the long term, and those who don't, comes down to mindset.

How we see ourselves in the mirror is vital to our well-being. If you see an overweight person in the mirror, whether it's the truth or not, it's your truth. People with this mindset are always *trying* to do better. Trying to lose weight, trying to make it to the gym, trying to make better choices. The problem with this is they are still embodying being an overweight person, and making decisions that overweight people would make.

Conversely, if what you see in the mirror is a fit person, then you will do things fit people do. Fit people make their health a priority. Fit people exercise on a regular basis. Fit people pay attention to the foods they eat and drink the most adult beverage in the world, water! Fit people find opportunities to be active and use their bodies in a variety of ways. Fit people are willing and able to say yes to the physical demands of life, mostly without reservation, because they view themselves as the type of person who can.

A fit mindset is no small task, and for those who were not fit growing up, this can be the last... and often most difficult... piece of the puzzle for a lifetime of healthy living. Whatever it takes to adopt this way of thinking, do it. Post-It notes on your mirror, daily reminders on your phone, a routine of daily affirmations and "I am" statements. All these things can make a difference and over time will shift your view towards knowing you're a fit human.

Success leaves clues. I'm not saying these are the only things that will make a person successful in their fitness journey, but I am saying that over two decades of coaching people has shown me those who do embrace these concepts are wildly more successful than those who don't.

I highly encourage you to follow suit and make good choices!

If you'd like to connect with me for coaching, for a conversation, for hilarious memes, or for the various shenanigans I continually put out in the world, please visit https://www.connectwithmarcz.com

Since 2003, Marc "The Fitness Ninja" Zalmanoff has been helping people live happier, healthier lives through improved fitness, nutrition, and mindset.

A gym owner in Frisco, Texas, Marc has a unique talent of blending science-based fitness and nutrition programming with empathetic coaching to meet people where they are, and help them achieve the results that have alluded them for far too long. Along with his never-ending wit and humor, Marc can help anyone who is ready for change.

Over the years Marc has realized being a business owner, regardless of the profession, requires an expanding skill set of personal growth, marketing, business skills, and a lot of written words. He knows people need to hear the right message in order to be moved to make positive changes in their lives.

Whether it's serving people in his gym, coaching people through his online programs, or educating and entertaining the masses on social media through his written content and memes, he is currently on a mission to Make America Fit Again and help people Make Good Choices, and will do whatever he can to make the biggest impact possible!

Marc currently resides in Frisco, Texas, with his beautiful wife Laura, his two boys, Marc and Cheech, and all his fur babies (Callie, Mary Jane, Ben, and Jim the Cat)!

CHAPTER SEVEN:
My Road To Redemption

By Mike Matli

This is my story how fitness has changed and, at times, saved my life. My journey started at the early age of twelve. My older cousin and his friends would lift weights at his house and after they would leave, I would try to copy what they did. My cousin was very athletic and the popular guy in school, so needless to say, I looked up to him. Being at that young age, I was also very influenced and a huge fan of WWF wrestling. Hulk Hogan was of course my favorite wrestler and I even had a Hulkamania workout set!

"Train, eat your vitamins, and say your prayers," as the Hulkster would say.

Throughout junior high school, I would lift with the stronger kids on the old circuit machine we had in a little back room, but it wasn't until high school that really changed and I was able to use an actual weight room. I was never a big kid in school, but I've always had the heart of a lion, even though my confidence never peaked in school.

I was a pretty shy kid, but once I was around the weights, that was my world. It was the one place where I didn't have to worry about anyone or their opinions. I took weightlifting classes every semester and during football season, I'd be the first one in and the last one out. This mentality has helped me in life to work for what I want with the ability to be a self-starter and need little or no supervision to complete the task. Even back then, I was very dedicated but I just didn't have the knowledge to grow.

Socially, the lifting didn't help my confidence grow until my senior year, but unfortunately, I was still a follower and that led me down the troubled path. During senior year, some of my friends got involved in the gang life and I followed suit. I suppose I wanted to feel like I belonged to something or had a purpose. I grew up with a loving and very supportive family but I guess this was me going against the grain. The thing with me is I have always put my all into everything I do, good or bad, and this time in my life it wasn't so good.

One night in June, two weeks after graduating from high school, I decided it was the night to prove my loyalty. Against the pleas of my best friend G, I went out with my other "friends" not knowing what the night had in store. All I knew was that they wanted me to drive since I had my own vehicle.

They had me take them to different spots and had me drop them off, and they would come back each time about ten minutes later. This went on for about four times, but the last time, a car pulled up to where I was, and they got out of the car and started handing me items out of that car.

Turns out, they were robbing people and even assaulted these last guys. We started to head home, when a police car started following us and turned its lights on, so I pulled over. As I did, the guy in the front seat put his pistol in my glove box. Before we knew it, there were about five police cars surrounding us with guns drawn. At eighteen years old and never having been in real trouble, I couldn't believe this was happening. I had just gotten accepted to Oklahoma State University and had the chance to play football. That was pretty much down the drain now.

This was the start of my downfall for the next decade. I ended up doing three months plus three years' probation for being an accessory to crime. Being incarcerated with grown men was definitely an eye opener, but best believe every time yard time was announced, I was out there hitting the weight pile. Weightlifting was my main purpose and I hadn't even realized it yet.

At this moment of my life, I was a lost soul and my biggest regrets were messing up my college admissions and embarrassing my family. From the ages of eighteen to around twenty-five, I couldn't keep myself out of trouble. I would be in and out of county jail for stupid decisions I made which usually involved drinking too much. Up until twenty, I had fallen off from working out and was more worried about running the streets.

I think not being dedicated in the gym went hand in hand with me going down this dark path, because at this time I really had no purpose. It wasn't until I was about twenty-five that I really started getting back into lifting weights, but my goal was for all the wrong reasons. Since my life just involved partying and clubbing, my intention was to get as swole as I could so people would look at me and say, *I do not want to get hit by that guy*, and it worked. I guess in my crazy world I thought I was earning respect.

Not until later would I learn how that really was done. When I was in the gym, I would push the heaviest weight I could. No technique, no proper nutrition, and definitely not enough rest. Just me taking my frustrations out on those weights and hoping not to injure myself.

For the next five years, I just really went with the flow, really taking anything that came my way. At age thirty, I was a bouncer at a bar downtown and soon was training mixed martial arts with one of the head bouncers, and we've remained good friends to this day. I really enjoyed that gig, but after a few months, I decided I really had to do something with my life to make decent money so I decided to get my CDL.

With my criminal record, I really had no choice. By this time, I had achieved an associate's degree in architectural drafting and also gotten certified as a personal trainer, but no one would hire me because of my past. This new journey in my life was a struggle as well. I basically started off at rock bottom. Making bottom dollar and living off the dollar menu just to survive.

Eventually things got better, and after I got used to spending four to six weeks on the road at a time, I brought my curl bar and a few weights on the truck with me. The road life was very stressful at times so my workouts at the end of my day kept me sane and really put me in a peaceful state of mind. Later in my driving days, I even bought a small grill so I would be able to do some food prep and start to eat healthy. I even started a YouTube channel trying to help fellow truck drivers with thirty-minute workout videos that could easily be done at the truck.

I was on the road for about six years when I got a local job delivering food service items. This job was very physical. During this time in 2012, my son was born, which totally changed my life forever. Now I wasn't just living for myself, but now I had someone who would be looking up to me. By now my confidence was at an all-time high, and I had learned the skills needed for the Alpha mentality and was no longer a follower but a leader.

One night in August of that year, G and I were hanging out with another friend from our school days at a local pool hall, and at the end of our night, we headed out to the parking lot, where a group of guys approached us. They evidently had a problem with our friend. As the argument got heated, three of them raised their shirts to show they had pistols in their waist bands. As I was trying to defuse the situation, my back got turned and I heard gunshots and my friend yelling that he had gotten hit. Without thinking, I jumped over him to cover him.

The cowards with the guns took off as I was trying to tend to my friend.

First responders showed up within minutes and transported him to the hospital, but they couldn't stop the bleeding, and he passed away that night. I think the only thing that kept me going back to my old self and seeking revenge was holding my son and realizing what I had to live for. My son literally saved my life in more ways than one.

After that tragic night, I really struggled with my emotions moving constantly from sadness to anger and rage. I would go to the gym consistently, but sometimes I couldn't finish because my emotions would get the best of me, and my mind would constantly relive those moments like a movie. I do think at the time, even though the workouts weren't the best at times, the consistency really helped me stay grounded as I would slowly move forward.

Finally, after about four years, what finally brought me a little peace was talking to G's father, and he told me to let it go and let God handle it.

By 2016, I was able to be motivated to do some positive things. I continued making videos for the truckers, because even in my not-so-good days, I always had a good heart and tried to help people and offer what knowledge I had. This was also when I started following Rich Piana, who had a huge impact on my life indirectly. I loved his hustle and how he always kept it real with the things he spoke about. He motivated me to create my gym apparel line, Stallion Squad Fitness. At this time, I also started helping people with programming and sample food plans.

I had the pleasure of meeting him in person at a meet and greet, and he signed a poster for my son. We spoke about meeting up at the Mr. Olympia competition, but, tragically, he passed away a month before that could happen.

By 2017, I was working locally and had a consistent gym schedule, and within two years, my bench went from 405 to 455 lbs. naturally. I was also learning more about technique and nutrition. When the Covid pandemic hit, luckily I had a setup at the house and was able to stay on my routine, and also created content in hopes of motivating people who watched my videos.

I pushed through the rest of the year and into the following year. At this time, I started to train at Flex Gym in Colorado Springs, Colorado. From the moment I walked through those doors, I was welcomed. The atmosphere was family-like, and this is where I decided I was going to compete as a powerlifting bench presser. I think being in this environment really helped me be a better person in my personal life as I was meeting some great people, and the two owners have been some of my biggest supporters.

My first meet was nerve wracking, but I achieved the state record for my division at 429 lbs. After that, I signed up for any meet I could make and traveled to Phoenix, Arizona, hitting 435 lbs. for my best lift and increasing my state record.

Then in 2021, I traveled to Tulsa, Oklahoma, but I failed at my 441 lbs. attempt. My son was along for that trip, and on the drive home, we had a talk about how failing isn't losing but is a learning experience to get better.

June came, and I competed in Denver, Colorado, where I hit 441 lbs. And along with increasing my state record, I also qualified for Nationals as it was an elite lift. My momentum stopped there, though, as in September I caught Covid and pneumonia, which put me down for about three weeks. On the fourth week, I came back determined but had literally lost all my strength. It took me about eight weeks to get back where I was strength-wise, but a month later, right before Christmas, I broke my right forearm. I just took this as another challenge and the chance to strengthen my left side. I did one-arm bench press on the Smith machine and other left sided dumbbell exercises for about six weeks until I was able to put pressure on my right arm again.

I could have felt sorry for myself, but what good would that have done? I've found that through all my years in the gym, it has helped me deal with failures in life and how to get through them by recognizing the problem and finding the solution.

I've come to learn a long time ago that life and the gym come hand in hand. As in life, you won't always have someone there to help you through a situation. You have to dig deep within yourself and fight through whatever situation is holding you down. Trust your own strength and conquer those obstacles in front of you. Don't be afraid of your failures as they will lead to your successes. I've done my best to teach my son these values since he was little.

After my recovery from injury, I trained for and competed in Nationals in Atlanta, Georgia. I was blessed enough to be able to bring my son along because it was here after only two years of competing, I accomplished my goal of breaking the world record for my division. My best lift was 457 lbs., which broke the record. For that moment, I felt like a superhero to my son and very proud of what I had accomplished. Honestly, my biggest motivation for chasing these records was to bring light back to my name in my grandfather's eyes before he passed away, and I think I accomplished that.

I enjoyed the taste of victory for a couple days, but after that it was back to business. Back in the gym, I started training for the next upcoming meet, which was in August in my hometown of Colorado Springs, but it didn't turn out so well. I only hit 441 lbs. and just had to take that loss.

There was no time to take off as the next meet was in November in Las Cruces, New Mexico. It was around September that I received one of the best emails I've ever gotten. I received an invitation to compete at the Mr.

Olympia competition in Las Vegas in December! This made my whole year! All my hard work was paying off.

At the competition in Las Cruces, I hit 463 lbs. and tied the National record. I have competed drug-free thus far, and I think that's what I'm most proud of in my late 40s. I was finally flying high again.

Being invited to the Mr. Olympia competition was something I couldn't have imagined five years prior. As I mentioned before, I go all out in everything I do. I think the average person may have quit with so many setbacks, but that's not what God put me here to do. Arriving at the Mr. Olympia competition for weigh ins, it really hit me. I'm was competing against world class lifters. It was surreal being in that atmosphere.

The next day starting warmups, I told myself, *"You made it, you fuckin' made it!"* I gave my all in my showing but failed on my last lift at 468 lbs. To my surprise, I won second place in my weight division! I was on cloud nine, especially since I competed drug free.

If you want something bad enough, put the work in and the results will speak for themselves.

Mike Matli has over thirty years of strength training experience, and last year he started offering his services as a strength coach both online and in person. Along with coaching, he also runs a gym apparel business, Stallion

Squad Fitness. which can be found at www.Stallionsquad.com

You can also join his the Facebook group, Stallion Squad Nation, for fitness tips and for any questions you may have.

CHAPTER EIGHT:
Fueling Your Passion for Fitness

By Alan Perez

The last fifteen years in the fitness industry has blessed me with amazing experiences. I've had the privilege of being able to coach numerous people with a broad variety of backgrounds, goals, and ambitions. Through those experiences, I have been fortunate enough to have learned many lessons that have been invaluable to my development, both personally and professionally.

Early in my career in fitness, I spent years developing fun and meaningful exercise programs for children with learning challenges. From there I transitioned into the rehab setting, working with clients recovering from specific challenges such as knee replacements, shoulder tears or spinal cord injuries. Years later I was developing a strong reputation at one of the biggest gym chains for consistently delivering amazing results for my clients. From there I decided to leave the large corporate gym space to create my own independent brand of Personal Training in Frisco, Texas. Today, I am building what I hope to be the best personal training studio in the Dallas area.

I've worked with and seen many fitness journeys. The pursuit of fitness is not easy. It is tough and challenging, and you'll be faced with many obstacles along the way. Even when everything is going well, long-term change requires an immense amount of time, consistency, and patience. My viewpoint regarding this reality is simple. If I am going to invest a lot of time, energy, and effort into my fitness, I might as well do it by choosing a meaningful activity that I can enjoy along my journey.

Finding Your Interest

Start with finding a fitness-related activity that genuinely interests you. Everyone usually thinks of fitness as going to the gym to lift weights and/or hopping on a treadmill. But really, fitness can be any type of physical activity that requires challenging yourself to improve your physical health. For some that interest might be running. For others it may be bodybuilding.

Or maybe it's something completely different like biking or even yoga. The point is that you must find what catches your eye and motivates you to dive deeper into that activity. There is something out there for everyone and you just have to be willing to think outside the box or "gym" if necessary. Personally, I love trying new fitness activities. I've done everything from swimming laps to salsa classes. In my case, I found the most joy from functional weight training, boxing, and indoor rock climbing.

Accountability

Seek accountability from the very beginning. An important recommendation I make to anyone on their fitness journey is to seek external help or guidance towards your goal. This can be anyone from a personal trainer to even a friend that takes walks with you around the neighborhood. I've had dozens of coaches and accountability partners over the years, and I wouldn't be the person I am today without them.

Having accountability in fitness is important because it can help you to stay motivated, make progress, and achieve your goals. People who have accountability in their fitness goals are considerably more likely to stick to their fitness routine. Having an accountability partner also provides an added layer of support and motivation. An accountability partner can help to keep you on track by regularly checking in with them, providing encouragement, and holding you accountable to your commitments. This can in turn help you to overcome obstacles and stay focused, even when faced with challenges or temptations to give up. Overall, having accountability in fitness can lead to increased motivation, better results, and improved physical and mental health.

Embrace the Struggle

Have the courage to show up to your fitness journey, not just physically, but mentally too. Show up with passion, determination, and the willingness to struggle through the learning phase of anything you choose to do. Of course, this is easier said than done. The learning phase of any activity you begin is always tough and requires patience. This is when managing your expectations comes in.

Managing your fitness expectations involves setting realistic, achievable goals and having a clear understanding of what you can expect from your fitness routine. It's important to remember that changes in physical fitness take time and effort, and progress may not always be linear.

Here are a few tips for managing your fitness expectations. First, set achievable goals. Start with small, achievable goals and gradually increase their difficulty as you make progress. Next, be patient. Physical changes take time, so be patient and allow yourself the necessary time to reach your goals. Along the way, I want you to celebrate the small victories.

Recognize and celebrate small successes along the way, such as reaching a new personal best or completing a challenging workout. Also don't forget to keep a record. Keeping track of your progress can help you stay motivated and see the improvements you've made over time.

Lastly, focus on what you can control. While external factors such as injury or illness may affect your progress, instead, focus on your effort and dedication. By managing your expectations and focusing on progress, you can enjoy the process and see the positive changes in your physical and mental health.

Become a New You

Be ready to significantly change your lifestyle to accommodate your fitness goal. Matching your lifestyle to your fitness goal involves aligning your daily habits, routines, and available resources with the desired outcome of your fitness regimen. This includes considering factors such as the amount of time and energy you can devote to physical activity, the types of exercise and equipment you have access to, and any dietary needs that you should strive for. The goal is to create a fitness plan that is sustainable and fits seamlessly into your lifestyle, rather than requiring major disruptions or sacrifices. And when you do have to make sacrifices to fit your fitness goal, you'll be filled with less stress and anxiety for doing so. This is due in part to how you've internalized the importance of your fitness routine. This then leads to a conscious acknowledgement of how essential exercise is to your life and therefore allowing yourself to continuously prioritize it.

Change if Necessary

There's something to be said about pushing through obstacles and jumping hurdles to get to your fitness goals. But sometimes, the passion and fun along the way just isn't there anymore. Sure, motivation is not something that will always be there. Discipline and consistency is what truly gets you where you want to be. But maybe there is a time when you really dig deep and conclude that this path or activity doesn't suit your needs any longer. I believe that it's at those times that you must really dig deep into your desires and figure out a different form of fitness that will keep pushing you forward.

Notice I didn't say to just abandon your fitness all together. I think that sometimes you just need to make a course adjustment along the way. This is where you see the beauty in how everyone has their own fitness journey. For example, maybe you picked up tennis a year ago and you've been having a wonderful time. But lately your knee has started acting up and it's painful to keep playing. Your doctor has suggested you quit and find a different activity that doesn't irritate it.

Or maybe you just don't enjoy the game anymore and you don't look forward to hitting the courts any longer. It's at times like these that I suggest it's perfectly healthy and to your advantage to seek a new fitness activity. It's your journey, and the most important thing is to find what works best for you and helps you maintain a consistent exercise routine.

Over the course of my career, I've seen these principles applied hundreds, if not thousands, of times. And I can personally attest to how life-changing they can be as I continue to grow in my own fitness journey too. Now, if there's one thing I'd like to remind you of is this: You don't have to wait until you reach your fitness goal to feel proud of how far you've come. As cliché as is it, the reward truly is in the journey, not the destination. I hope for you to experience your fitness journey to its fullest and enjoy your amazing accomplishments along the way.

If you would like to connect with me, ask questions about my coaching services, or just share your fitness journey with me, contact me at alanperezfitness@gmail.com

Alan Perez specializes in catering to individuals who are seeking expert guidance in personal training, injury prevention and nutrition guidance. Alan has maintained a thriving personal training business for over a decade and is a highly regarded trainer in the North Dallas, Texas, community. He has also maintained an extensive amount of education in areas such as spine health, post-rehab shoulder/knee exercise, and nutritional coaching. Alan has helped hundreds of clients with a primary focus on injury prevention and recovery with his unique and personalized programs.

CHAPTER NINE:
To Be Resilient – As Created By Your Health And Fitness

By David Rohland

I find it so interesting how some days just start like any other day. It was July 2018 and I just started our grill to get ready for dinner. I came back in the house and my wife Melissa was on the phone. At that time, I had been married for almost thirty years. When you're with someone for that long, you certainly get an innate sense as to something being wrong.

I could feel it as soon as I walked in the door. She was on the phone, looked at me, and mouthed the word *cancer*. You know those moments. Everything stops. Blood rushes to your ears. And you're quickly trying to make some sense of what's going on.

Yes, that was the moment when we received a call from the oncologist, informing us that my beautiful wife had breast cancer. This was confounding to me, as just a few days prior we were told that the tumor that they found, and removed, was benign. How could this be? We were told she was fine; Where did it go wrong?

Let me back up a little bit. Early in 2018, Melissa found a lump on her breast. She went in for the exam and they told her that it was "nothing." But as a few weeks went on, I think Melissa knew that something was not right. She went back and had it checked again. "Nothing."

A few more weeks went by, and Melissa felt as though the lump was growing. A surgery date was set to remove the lump. I remember being in the waiting room post-surgery. Her doctor came out and said, "Mr. Rohland, everything looks great. I've been doing this for a long time and I am eighty percent sure that this is not cancer. No, let me say, ninety-five percent sure that this is not cancer." And then, just a few days later, we receive *that call* letting us know that the tumor was indeed cancerous.

Melissa was diagnosed with stage 2, triple negative, breast cancer. For the uneducated like me… that's pretty bad. Chemotherapy, surgeries, radiation, lots of praying, and much love from family and friends.

Watching my wife go through chemo was brutal. And I am not trying to compare my perspective to what she was going through. I had been a gym junkie for years. In fact, Melissa and I met in a gym, as cliché as that sounds. One day, deep into the chemo treatments, Melissa told me to go to the gym!

"I can't go to the gym. I can't leave your side." She said, "I *need* you at your very best. I need you at your strongest and healthiest. I need you to be taking care of yourself."

Take the time to care for yourself so that you can best care for your loved ones and those that are depending upon you.

I believe it was at that point that "going to the gym" became so much more about the mental aspects versus the physical aspects. She was right (as happens quite often). I had to take that time to clear my head so that I could help her with her recovery.

As I reflect back upon that time, there is not a doubt in my mind that the end of the story would be very different if Melissa had not taken such accountability for her own health and fitness. In fact, I believe that Melissa found the lump simply because she was in good shape leading up to that moment.

Take accountability for your own health and fitness—No one is coming to your rescue.

For me, there is a real lesson to be learned here: We all need to be our own self-advocate for our health, because no one is coming to our rescue!

Let me jump to the end of the story… Melissa is now almost five years cancer free, doing great, and I would say healthier than ever! And that is all because she takes accountability for and being an advocate of her own health! Chemo is crazy on the body, and Melissa will tell you that proper nutrition and consistent weight training have been key to her recovery.

She and I have three amazing children who are now young men. And watching Melissa go through this with such grace has been a real learning lesson for all of us. There is no quit! And tomorrow holds no guarantees.

Health and fitness has given me—taught me—the resiliency to handle all that life throws at me.

For me, how can I not hit the gym hard and take care of myself after seeing all that she went through? But "lifting heavy things" is just a part of the equation. At that time, all our efforts were about getting rid of the cancer. I don't think we were properly prepared for "getting rid of the chemo." This is where proper nutrition really came into play.

Every morning post-chemo, I would come downstairs and find Melissa at our kitchen table wringing her hands together in pain. The slightest bump would send pain through her body. Was it the cancer? Chemo? Other? Just getting older? How long would this last? Forever? It was so hard to watch, and absolutely, heart-breaking.

We tackled this with a strategy and discovered that the pain was largely nutrition-based. Over time, we discovered the food items that worked for her and the ones that didn't work. We needed to be careful. We needed to be diligent. It also made us very aware of the foods we ate and what we put into our bodies. Additionally, this created an environment in which I wanted to dig deeper and further educate myself on the nutrition aspect of health, fitness, and wellness!

We can get so focused on our families and busy lives that we slowly get desensitized as to what makes us feel good.

I believe that we can have it all. Perhaps we can't have everything at the exact same time, but we can have it all. I worked for thirty-three years, in corporate America, traveling the United States, while raising three children with my wife who also has a demanding career. I understand the challenges of busy adulthood.

Even through my various responsibilities and travels while I was working in corporate America, it was important for me to stay focused on my personal health and fitness. In 1999, I received an honorable mention award in a body composition challenge. In 2000, I earned my black belt in martial arts. And I taught a weekly boot camp-style class for years. The friendships and knowledge developed through these relationships and programs have been profound, and I've grown tremendous confidence to be able to step out and help others.

There are times when we need to focus on that new job, or we are preparing to move into the new house, or we are getting ready for the new baby. There are also times when we can better focus on our health and fitness. I love to work with my people and adopt a variety of "training blocks" to help them navigate all the seasons of their life. We all have the ability to best prepare ourselves for everything that is coming our way: the blessings, as well as the challenges.

The varied dynamics of my life have led me to develop tools to aid in accomplishing my mission, including time management, scheduling, focusing on the right priorities at the right time, and giving ample time to loving the moments.

When people ask me why I train, I often say, *Because I can,* or I say, *For those that can't —and want to.* I mean that because there was a time in which I really questioned if I would be able to do many of the things that I love so much because of physical challenges. And, I have dear friends who suffered from terrible diseases and were unable to train.

The one BIG thing that I learned over these past few years is to *Seize the Day*, because we don't know what tomorrow will bring! And, with this thought in mind, I left corporate America in November 2019. I considered myself retired for the few months prior to the pandemic.

Then in July 2020, after much thought, I decided to follow my passion and start my own business. I wanted to take my love for fitness, nutrition, and coaching to the next level by helping others achieve their health, fitness, and lifestyle goals. Oddly enough, the pandemic gave me the idea to begin Today's Warrior. The quarantine gave me the time to hit the books, focusing on my nutritional and training courses of study.

I truly enjoy helping people establish healthy and realistic goals, evaluate their nutrition, make nutritional recommendations based upon their goals, current habits and lifestyle, and develop training programs. I enjoy helping others with their mind-set and accountability, and to make this work for them within their life and unique individual environment.

If you are struggling with your own health and fitness while trying to wear the many hats that we are required to wear, I hope that you will reach out to me. If you know anyone that is struggling with cancer—including their caregivers—I do have additional information on my YouTube page. Until then…

I hope that you will take a little time every day to focus on YOU so that you can be at your best for all of those depending on you.

David Rohland is a Certified Personal Trainer and Nutrition Specialist residing in Central Pennsylvania. Focusing on maximizing the potential of others through training, education, mentoring, and support services, during all seasons of life, David's goal is to leave a legacy for his family to be proud of, and to impact the lives of others in a positive way.

david@todayswarriorcoaching.com
Today's Warrior - Home (todayswarriorcoaching.com)
https://www.facebook.com/groups/realhealthandfitnesstalkfor todaysbusyadults/

CHAPTER TEN:
Questions, Questions and More Questions

By Martin Higgins

Let me tell you a story of a nerd… that's me by the way.

But before I do, a spoiler…

My approach to health and fitness is, perhaps, unconventional. It evolved out of necessity, curiosity, and a deep down need to do things right. It started with science and then became scientific (and as you'll see, those things aren't entirely the same). Just because an idea is generally accepted, doesn't make it true. Just because a method works for some people, that doesn't make it work for everyone. For every puzzle (and human health is really a set of puzzles to solve), I question, I dig, I verify and I evaluate.

Onto my story.

Every story has a beginning somewhere and mine began as a kid who loved to read. I had my nose in a book the whole time. Everything science from how the universe works to subatomic particles and (slightly larger) how our cells work. I was a proper nerdy kid.

When I wasn't reading or otherwise nerding out, I'd be playing in the woods: making dens, catching newts, making camp fires, riding bikes, and all the other things that make up a childhood full of adventure. Later those adventures just got bigger with canoe trips lasting many days, climbing mountains in all corners of the world, desert treks (both scorching and frozen), and anything else that caught my imagination. Science was my belief system and everything I did was explainable in science.

And therein lies a small glitch. Some of the science during all this time just didn't quite sit right with me. There were things I'd been taught in school that I just didn't quite understand. Mostly these things were in the biology classes but they cropped up in a few other places as well. My assumption was that I was cut out for the more mathematical sciences around physics rather than the less clearly defined ones such as biology and psychology.

That assumption later proved to be incorrect but not for a reason I expected or could have predicted at the time.

Several things came about that shook my scientific viewpoint. Call them little epiphanies if you like. Call them waking up. Call them finding something more. Whatever you call them, the result was the same. Science stopped being neat and tidy and easily pinned down under the weight of numbers.

The Injury

There I was kayaking through the Mexican jungle. It was day thirteen of an expedition. It was a Friday. It was also the day after I nearly died.

Our intrepid team were there to paddle some high-spirited rivers and on Thursday, we had revisited one exciting section from a couple of days before. There had been a storm in between and the river was somewhat bouncier than it had been previously. I tried to miss a big stopper (because it was the unfriendly sort that tries to eat you up, chew you around a while, and then slowly digests you). I failed. I got thoroughly pounded for a while. My friend Sam had time to get out of his boat, clamber up the bank alongside where I was, and assess that there was nothing he could do to help. I got 'washing-machined' long enough to run out of air and start to get some oxygen from the frothy water around me. My subconscious kicked in and I pulled the escape of the century by rolling up (not that I knew which way up was), surfing to the edge and then applying PLF (Paddle Like, err, Very Hard) out of the side to safety.

But that's not the science problem.

On the Friday a Grade 5 rapid called The Brain decided to twitch me, invert me, and rip my arm out of its socket. The team did a sterling job getting my arm back in its socket so I was able to bash my way out of the jungle, back to the truck, back to the airport and back home to the United Kingdom. Still no issues with science.

I got my dislocation checked out and was allocated a physiotherapist by the healthcare system. This is where science got shaky. The physio (a trade based on relatively simple biomechanics) gave me exercises which were meant to improve my shoulder but were exactly the wrong things to do.

They made it worse. The physio was supposed to know her stuff. I did my own research, found the issue, and fixed it myself. At that point, science was shown not to be trusted quite as completely.

The Pain

Roll the clock forwards a few years and I was getting some pain in my knee. It was in one of my periods of software consultancy work with many hours spent behind a desk. Many hours spent teaching classes. Many hours in trains, planes and automobiles… My knee hurt like crazy any time I spent more than about a half-hour in any one position. I did the sensible thing and went to a doctor and then a physio for assessment. The first physio gave me some exercises and said I'd need orthotics. He didn't sound very sure, so I went to another. The second physio said the same (but a bit clearer). Expensive orthotics and lots of exercises. Still a little unsure, I went to a third who also did gait analysis. He also recommended orthotics and also showed me some fancy foot strike and plantar images indicating I had flattened arches. I was told it's impossible to recover a flattened arch so being propped up is the only option.

None of this sat well for me so I started doing some more reading. I was into my trail running then and I read Born to Run. That book really opened my eyes but it also led me down some rabbit holes. My first decision was to stop wearing shoes or only very minimal ones and to start training my feet and legs to cope with the switch to a barefoot approach. That was the end of my knee problems.

The Weight Loss

The other thing I unearthed was a hint towards some new diet ideas which I did some more digging into. That led me down various paths resulting in a weight drop of forty-two lbs. in five weeks which have stayed off permanently. This was awesome because I'd always assumed my weight was a genetic thing and I would never be particularly trim. It was also another shake to my scientific mind as this deep dive into nutrition, cell behaviours, and ultimately the world of science as a whole, left me questioning pretty much everything I'd read or been taught before.

The Discovery

I'd discovered that some of the basic principles I had been taught formally were based on information which was driven by ends other than the pure and unadulterated quest for truth.

Many questions were left unanswered in the science or the answers were clearly wrong. There were questions which were ignored in the literature purely because there was no recorded evidence or no method of measurement for them.

Many of the concepts I unearthed would go against the established science I knew to be 'true'. Many also worked really well in practice. On top of that they made sense to me. It wasn't just that they 'seemed to work' for me but also that they felt like truth. I suppose you could say I 'found science'. Not the science of my youth filled with neat formulae placed in clearly defined boxes, but the science filled with pieces that clicked into place with other scientific jigsaw pieces. This was the science that required questioning rather than being blindly followed. The science that runs along at the grass roots of how everything is rather than how we'd like it to be.

So now my scientific mind is one of curiosity. It is also one of mistrust. Not mistrust in terms of assuming that everything I read is untrue. This is mistrust it terms of reading something, doing some further research to confirm that it is valid, and also running it by my litmus test of 'does it feel like the truth'?

The Outcome

Then the burning question to all of this is, What's this got to do with health, fitness and adventure coaching?

Well, it's led me to the development of my Six Core Elements To Thriving Without Limits. These are the backbone of human wellbeing and peak performance.

The Six Core Elements are:

Nutrition

Perhaps the single most misunderstood and misinformed area of human health. Most health professionals try to put a spin on what you should or shouldn't eat and drink, forgetting for the most part that each person has their own unique requirements. There are some basic, and often ignored, truths of how your cells work and interact, and then it's down to your unique makeup as to what is best. Science first, then the human element and a sprinkling of personalisation and flexibility on the top.

Strength

Like nutrition, strength attracts a wild array of distorted truth: *You should do this fancy exercise and it'll make you a superhuman in under five minutes a day without breaking a sweat.* Unfortunately, it doesn't work like that either. The simple version of the truth is that to get your body to change you need to give it a reason to do so. If you want to be more capable, more able to complete everything you plan for each day, then you need to demonstrate to your body what this entails.

Movement

Movement allows your body to perform actions wherever and whenever you need it to. Lifting a box is one thing, placing it on a high shelf needs the ability to stretch to that shelf. Picking up your kids means you need to be able to bend down. Running to catch a bus means you need to be able to run: your joints need to move, your heart and lungs need to perform their tasks properly, you need to not fall over. Movement is about making sure your body can actually move.

Nature

Humans are biological systems. We spent over three million years evolving and functioning within natural environments. It's only really the last few hundred years that we have had to try to fit into urban environments. As biological systems operating in natural environments we have developed an affinity for how nature interacts with us. We get to relax in nature. Our stresses dissolve. Our minds and bodies can heal. We don't get sick as much. In short, we thrive in nature but only barely survive without it.

Adventure

Adventure is an oft forgotten element of human health. Throughout human history we have developed many integral functions within the brain that thrive on the push that challenging activities give us. In the earlier days, those activities were about survival: getting away from predators, accessing nests and hives to get food, and all the other things humans had to do to stay alive. In modern times many of these challenges have gone away as the basics of survival were covered by societies and systems. That left an actual gap in how we work, which was steadily replaced by other things. Adventure can mean many things. It can be the challenge of racing, the excitement of adrenalin sports, the wonder of going to remote places, and the progression of exploration. Our brains need these triggers, so adventure in its many guises has become a vital part of our mental health.

Rest

When we rest, our bodies and our minds can sort out what we need for the next day. Without rest, there is no repair or development. Without rest, there is no ordering of information or solidifying what we've learnt. Without rest, we don't gain all of the benefits from our training, learning, and adventures. Our gains may be triggered by our activities but the gains themselves occur during rest.

Simply put, I now have the skills and the knowledge to solve problems. Some people come to me who may have 'tried everything' to lose weight. Not only do I help them with that goal but leave them able to continue for the rest of their lives. Some people come to me wanting to do well in a big challenge like climbing a mountain, running a marathon, or completing an Ironman triathlon. They invariably outperform their original goals and go on to even more besides. Some people come to me with pain that just won't go away and I help them reduce the pain and it often goes away completely.

All because I question everything…

If you've read through my story, you already have a fair idea of who and what I am. What I am, of course, is a nerd with a difference. I'm a nerd in the sense that I have a deep love and understanding of all things science. I'm also a nerd in the sense that I'm on the smarter end of the IQ scale (I'm not bragging—it's just true). Where I differ from most nerds though is that I also love being in nature, being active, and being the best I can be for myself, my family, and those who choose to ask for my help.

If you're looking purely at my qualifications, then you'll find a good selection of advanced subjects from the areas of health, nutrition, coaching, fitness, adventure sports, and leadership. If you're looking at my experience, it spans over three decades of professional activity in these fields (plus the time I indulged my passions in my school years).

If you want to find out a little more about me, what I do, and perhaps how I can help you solve your own health, fitness, and adventure related puzzles, and move you on to a better life, then find me on my Facebook page @martinhigginscoaching or my website www.martinhigginscoaching.com

About The Authors

Jonathan Lautermilch is the CEO of Smart Shark, a highly sought-after business integration consultancy. and Co-Founder of Fit Pro Collective, a business mastermind for fitness professionals. Jonathan's mission in life is to help business owners turn their vision into reality.

Jonathan has 14 years of business development experience, is a best-selling author, and is a Co-Host on the Real Talk With Real Fit Pros Podcast. Jonathan has coached thousands of coaches and business owners in starting, scaling, and growing their businesses. He's also a loving husband, and a soon-to-be father and lives in Dallas, Texas.

Since 2003, **Marc "The Fitness Ninja" Zalmanoff** has been helping people live happier, healthier lives through improved fitness, nutrition, and mindset.

A gym owner in Frisco, Texas, Marc has a unique talent of blending science-based fitness and nutrition programming with empathetic coaching to meet people where they are, and help them achieve the results that have alluded them for far too long. Along with his never-ending wit and humor, Marc can help anyone who is ready for change.

He is currently on a mission to Make America Fit Again and help people Make Good Choices, and will do whatever he can to make the biggest impact possible!

Marc currently resides in Frisco, Texas, with his beautiful wife Laura, his two boys, Marc and Cheech, and all his fur babies (Callie, Mary Jane, Ben, and Jim the Cat)!

www.ingramcontent.com/pod-product-compliance
Lightning Source LLC
Chambersburg PA
CBHW051756250726
48659CB00001B/456